Interm

MW00937072

16/8

Delicious Recipes & Meal Plan for 3 Weeks

Lose Weight with the Innovative Intermittent Fasting 16/8 Method

By Jason Cooper

Disclaimer

Table of Contents

Introduction

The world of weight loss and overall health and wellbeing is a confusing one. It seems that every single week there is a new fad diet on the block, or another addition to something which we thought we had mastered the understanding of! Who said being healthy was easy?

For anyone who has weight to lose, it's important to find the right type of diet to suit your needs. In many ways the 'right' kind of diet won't be a diet at all, it will be a lifestyle change which helps you lose weight, become healthier, and sustain it all in the end.

It seems that the low carbohydrate, high fat combination lifestyle change is a popular one at the moment, but that doesn't work for everyone. Having to count carbs, protein, and make sure you're eating enough fat content can be too time consuming, and it's also not so easy to incorporate this kind of eating regime and general lifestyle change into your routine.

There is another option.

Have you heard of intermittent fasting?

The word 'fasting' puts many people off, but this new routine is far easier than you might think, and it actually yields some very beneficial effects on your health; of course, one of those benefits is weight loss.

This book is designed for anyone who wants to become healthier, have more energy, turn back the ticking clock of aging, as well as anyone who wants to lose weight and maintain a healthy number on the scales afterwards. We'll first talk about what intermittent fasting is, as well as exploring the many benefits. Of course, we want to give you all the information possible, and that means both sides of the coin; in that regard we'll cover a few of the possible downsides too. If you have all information available to you, you can make an informed decision as to the best way forward for you.

If you do an online search into the various different types of intermittent fasting, you'll see a long list of methods. This book isn't going to give you a huge amount of choice and confess the matter further, it's going to give you the easiest to follow, the easiest to incorporate into your lifestyle method, and that is the 16:8 method. We will talk about the other methods just for completeness' sake, but the 16:8 is certainly the method we would choose if we were going to make a decision. You'll see why when we get into more detail, but because we have to give you all the facts, because we're responsible information givers, and you're an adult who can make their own mind up, you'll find a chapter dedicated to the other intermittent fasting methods, as well as their pros and cons.

At the end of the book we'll also give you a bonus chapter, a gift from us to you, if you will! This is 20 delicious and easy to make recipes which will easily fit into your new 16:8 lifestyle, whether you choose to make them on a regular basis or not. The idea is that you can see how easy this lifestyle is to follow, and how it really doesn't restrict you in any way at all. All you need to do is eat healthier and try new things as a result. That's not so hard, especially when you start to feel the benefits coming your way. Weight loss and general health and well-being has a habit of being quite addictive once you feel it!

If this all sounds a little confusing at this point, don't worry. Everything will become abundantly clearly as you make your way through this book, and as your understanding grows. At the same time, your excitement should grow too!

Now, sit back and relax. You're about to embark on a journey towards total health and wellbeing, and it's far easier than you might think.

Chapter 1: What is Intermittent Fasting?

For as long as humans have roamed the Earth, there has been fasting. Sometimes we don't realize we're fasting, sometimes we do, but fasting has always been there.

Fasting doesn't cause bad health. Fasting does not cause death. Fasting is not dangerous. Cavemen and cavewomen fasted because of a lack of food and a need to preserve, many religious practices encourage fasting, such as the Muslim Holy month of Ramadan, and during Lent in Christianity. Put simply, fasting isn't something out of the ordinary, and the human body is more than capable of going without food for a short amount of time. Your body naturally fasts during your sleeping time at night!

Before we begin, you need to banish the idea that fasting is dangerous out of your mind. Fasting is safe, provided you follow the rules and eat when you're supposed to. There is a very big difference between fasting and starving. When you attempt to starve yourself, you're doing so because you are choosing not to eat. This is dangerous and comes with a myriad of serious health concerns attached to it.

Warning aside, let's delve a little deeper into the world of intermittent fasting and explain exactly what it is.

Intermittent fasting, as the name suggests, is fasting intermittently throughout the day. It is a cycle of eating and fasting, and the plus point is that there are no rules in terms of what you can eat and what you can't, provided you stick to healthy in general. For this reason, intermittent fasting is the eating pattern of choice. You can still enjoy the odd bar of chocolate if you want to, but you need to ensure you stick to moderation and that you do so within your eating window only. Basically, intermittent fasting doesn't tell you what to eat, it tells you when to eat it.

Whilst many so-called diets are restrictive in terms of social life, e.g. you may struggle to go out for a meal with friends because you're worried about overeating, intermittent fasting doesn't come with that problem attached. You can go out, provided you schedule it for your eating window, and you can eat what you want, within reason. Obviously, you can't go around eating three pizzas simply because there are no rules, but a couple of slices is fine!

There are many different types of intermittent fasting, and the only major difference between them is when you can eat. There are no rules in terms of what you can eat; these types all allow you to eat at different times, or different quantities of time. For instance, some might advocate a full day of fasting, perhaps twice per week, whilst others will simply ask you to fast for x number of hours every day. In this case, you need to pick the type which suits your lifestyle best. This book is going to cover the 16:8 intermittent fasting type, and in our next chapter we're going to give you the low down on what that means. For now, you simply need to know that this is probably the easiest intermittent fasting method around, and it's also arguably the most popular as a result.

The most common question about intermittent fasting is about hunger. Surely, you'll be super-hungry during your fasting times? Actually, no! You can still drink water, unsweetened, black tea and coffee, and any other drinks which contain no calories when you're fasting, and this is often enough to do away with any slight hunger pangs you might feel. Obviously when you first start fasting, you're going to notice a little in the way of hunger, but this is just a sign that your body needs to get used to your new routine.

Most people report that once they are established within their intermittent fasting method, they do not notice hunger, and usually have more energy when they're fasting! Strange, but true.

What Happens to The Body During a Fast?

The reason that intermittent fasting is so popular, or IF, as you might hear it referred to, is because of the health benefits, as well as the boost to weight loss.

When you refrain from eating for even a short while, many different routine bodily processes change. This is because your body suddenly things 'hang on a minute, where's the food?', and starts to panic that nothing else is going to be forthcoming. This kickstarts processes which actually help the body to thrive and survive in such circumstances. These processes all have to do with genes, cellular repair systems, and hormones, which also give you extra energy as a result.

Blood sugar and insulin (a hormone which is associated with weight gain) reduce quite drastically, and the fat burning switch is turned firmly on. This means that you're actually burning fat for energy, rather than carbohydrates, which are the usual first port of call for the body. Calories are also restricted naturally, simply because you're having more time when you're not eating (fasting), and that in itself leads to weight loss. Of course, this does mean you have to be careful you're not overeating during your eating window.

We're going to cover the benefits of intermittent fasting shortly, but in terms of what happens within your body, you're basically creating a calorie deficit which lends itself towards weight loss, whilst kick-starting metabolic processes within the body that help your energy levels, and your general wellbeing.

All in all, intermittent fasting is a major win-win!

The Benefits of Intermittent Fasting

There are many science-based benefits of intermittent fasting which certainly put a boost towards following a one of the methods available. The main benefits are shown below.

- **May help to increase sensitivity to insulin** - When insulin levels are too high, all manner of rather unpleasant effect occurs, such as obesity for one. Most chronic diseases are linked to some form of insulin resistance or sensitivity, so the ability to reduce the chances of this occurring means less chance of chronic diseases too!

- **Helps normalize leptin and ghrelin levels** - These are two hormones which are responsible for telling you when you've eaten enough, e.g. you're full, and telling you when you're hungry in the first place. When these two hormones are all over the place, you're likely to eat when you don't need to, and you're likely to overeat and therefore gain weight. There are many reasons these two hormones can be out of whack, but intermittent fasting has been shown to help normalize levels, so you naturally know when to stop eating and you naturally know when you are actually hungry.

- **Can lower bad cholesterol levels, by reducing triglycerides** - There is good cholesterol in the body (HDL) and there is bad (LDL). Triglycerides help increase the amount of bad cholesterol within the body, which is linked to heart disease, blocked arteries, heart attacks, and stroke, as a few rather worrying examples. Intermittent fasting can help to reduce the number of triglycerides, and therefore reduce the amount of bad cholesterol in your system.

- **Increases the HGH hormone within the body** - This hormone is quite important if you want to lose weight, because it is known widely as the 'fitness hormone'. This hormone ensures overall health and wellbeing, but it also does a lot to increase your metabolism. Metabolism is the rate at which you burn fat, amongst other functions, and the higher this rate, the more weight you will lose! Increasing this hormone is therefore vital if you want to slim down, but it also helps you to build muscle too, when used in conjunction with weight bearing exercise. Again, this is important because the leaner muscle you have, the more fat you will burn, and the faster you will burn it.

- **Reduces the amount of inflammation within the body** - Inflammation is responsible for a hung number of conditions and occurs when the body is put under undue stress.

Of course, we're led to believe that inflammation is good, because it protects injuries and ensures we heal. That's true, but when these levels remain high for a long period of time, this inflammation can be damaging. Lower levels of inflammation are connected with overall good health and intermittent fasting can help you achieve that.

- **Helps to boost renewal of cells and their function** - There is a metabolic process called 'autophagy' which happens when the body is fasting. This is because the body automatically thinks it's going to starve, but of course, that's not the case! When you search a little deeper into what autophagy is, it can seem a little terrifying, because it's literally the body eating itself. Now, don't panic! When this happens, the body is consuming and ridding itself of old cells, damaged cells, and any which simply don't live up to the mark. What is left behind is fresh, new, and all-powerful cells which have the habit of helping your body function are more effectively, but also make you look younger too!

- **Ensures the body burns fat, rather than carbs** - When you're following a regular diet, your body will automatically go to the carbs you consume as its first port of call for energy. This means that any existing fat cells just stay there, untouched, and probably growing. When your body is forced to burn fat instead, because carbs are scarce or because you're fasting, it switches to fats instead. This means existing fat stores are quickly eaten up, resulting in weight loss, and it also means that you need to eat a diet which is higher in fat, in order to satisfy your body's burning needs. Fat is far more satiating than regular low-calorie options, which of course means less hunger. It's win-win!

- **Many helps to reverse type II diabetes** - There is some suggestion that intermittent fasting may help to reverse type II diabetes and can also help to prevent it too. Of course, not every single person who suffers from type

II diabetes is going to find a total reversal and cure in intermittent fasting, but it may certainly help to manage blood sugar and insulin levels, which in itself aids in the management of the condition.

- **Boosts the immune system** - Intermittent fasting has been shown to boost the function of the immune system, ensuring that you don't fall foul of every single cold, 'flu, and virus that is doing the rounds. By boosting your immune function you are also helping with your overall gut health, as the majority of your immune system is actually situated in your stomach!

- **May help to lower blood pressure** - Intermittent fasting may also naturally lower blood pressure levels, which helps to reduce the risk of heart disease, heart attack, and stroke. Anyone who is taking regular medication for blood pressure should continue to do so and see their doctor for regular blood pressure readings, but for anyone who naturally wants to reduce their levels, intermittent fasting has been shown to be very useful indeed.

- **May reduce the risk of developing certain types of cancer** - Whilst intermittent fasting should never be considered an avoidance tactic for cancer development, the way fasting affects the cells, and the fact that you are taking away certain types of food which cancerous cells feed on, means that your risk of developing cancer (certain types) is far lower. Of course, you're living a healthier lifestyle, which also helps!

- **May help you live longer** - One of the commonly heard benefits of intermittent fasting is that it may help you live for longer. Whilst it's probably not going to see you into your 100s, intermittent fasting may help with longevity, provided it is combined with a generally healthy lifestyle and plenty of exercise. There are many reasons why this is the case, including insulin sensitivity normalization, and general slowing of the aging process.

- **Helps with brain function and helps to protect against age-related brain conditions** - Intermittent fasting has been shown to help people concentrate and focus far easier, helping with cognitive function overall. In addition, intermittent fasting may give some protection against age-related diseases of the brain and neurological system, including Alzheimer's, Parkinson's, and dementia. This is all down to something called ketones, which are produced naturally by the body during fat burning.

Of course, the main reason why people tend to look towards intermittent fasting in the first place is because they want to lose weight, and we haven't mentioned that as a benefit. Of course it is one, but we need to highlight the potential health benefits too! When you embark on an intermittent fasting lifestyle, provided you eat when you're supposed to and you don't go completely crazy on the carbs and calories during your eating window, weight loss is practically guaranteed.

The biggest reason why people stick with intermittent fasting in the long term is not only because of the weight loss and the extra energy, but it's also about how easy it is to fit into your regular lifestyle. Low calorie and fad diets are difficult to sustain, simply because they're far too restrictive and they don't give you any wiggle room, especially when it comes to your social life. As we get into the how's and why's of the 16:8 intermittent fasting method, our method of choice, you'll begin to see far more clearly why this type of eating habit is so popular - you don't have to restrict yourself, and if you want to head out for a meal with friends, you can certainly do so!

The Potential Downsides of Intermittent Fasting

Everything in life has pros and cons, and because we believe in being transparent and complete, allowing you to make a decision that is based on all the information and not just some of it, it's important to point out the possible downsides of intermittent fasting too.

The biggest downside of intermittent fasting is that you do need to fast for some of the day in order to make it work! That is the deal! The good thing about the 16:8 method, as you will come to find out, is that you can easily stretch that to ensure that you're sleeping for most of it, so it is far less noticeable. You can also move your fasting period to the times which suit you. It doesn't matter when you fast, provided you follow the rules and fast for the right amount of time consecutively.

Of course, fasting will make you hungry at first. This is also something you can't avoid. Over time, the non-hungry plus point will kick in, but at first, you're likely to notice pangs. These might also be quite severe at first, but you will find ways to deal with them, such as distraction techniques, delayed gratification, and drinking water. Much of the time, when we think we're hungry we're actually not; we're normally just bored, or even thirsty. Taking a drink of water, or even having a cup of unsweetened, black tea or coffee is allowed during your fasting periods, and this can take the edge off any hunger pangs you're feeling.

The biggest challenge that most people face when starting the intermittent fasting lifestyle is not overeating during their eating window. When you've been fasting for x number of hours, you're going to be hungry by the time your eating window starts. This can mean that you're quite open to grabbing the biggest meal around, no matter what it contains. Remember, intermittent fasting doesn't tell you what you can and can't eat, but you do still need to eat healthily. There is no diet on this planet that will let you eat chips, pizza, chocolate, and all the sugary, carb-laden treats you normally crave, because these are duty-bound towards weight again! You can have the odd treat when following intermittent fasting, but the will power you need to develop stops you from overindulging when your fast finishes.

You will probably also come to quickly realize that if you overindulge after a fast, your stomach is going to tell you very loudly and possibly quite spectacularly that it doesn't approve! Having a meal which is too heavy after a fast can lead to stomach aches, gas, and upsets. It's best to stick with light foods and build up over time. Developing will power and knowing the difference between healthy foods and terrible foods will be something you learn quite quickly, but the fact that nothing is restricted can often mean those with less self-discipline can fall foul of this biggest of intermittent fasting pitfalls.

There are also a few concerns about women finding it harder to complete intermittent fasting, compared to women. This is all down to hormones. Women are far more sensitive to calorie fluctuations than men, because women have different hormones. This means that when calories are restricted, hormone levels change. When hormone levels change, side effects can occur. The good news is that the 16:8 method we're going to talk about is one of the best intermittent fasting methods for women, because it doesn't affect hormones to a great degree. Some other methods i.e. types which ask you to fast for a full day, a few times per week, are far more likely to cause hormonal disturbances for women. For the most part, you can manage any side effects by choosing the right method.

A Word of Caution

Intermittent fasting isn't for everyone, just as any change in lifestyle isn't for everyone too. If you have any pre-existing medical conditions or you're on any type of medication, it's best to have a chat with your doctor and inform him or her what you're thinking of trying. In this case you will either get the green light to go ahead, or you will be advised against it. Always listen to your doctor and take their advice.

For the most part however, there are few people who aren't suitable to follow intermittent fasting, especially the 16:8 method. Pregnant women are advised not to follow intermittent fasting, and instead wait until after the baby is born. If you're breastfeeding, speak to your doctor about your calorie requirements and whether or not this is a suitable option for you. Again, always listen to their advice and take it seriously.

It's also vitally important that you ensure you eat when you are supposed to. If you fast and then don't break the fast, e.g. you don't start to eat when you're allowed, you're effectively shifting the focus from fasting to starving, and we've already established that is NOT A GOOD THING. Your body requires a certain amount of nutritional amount every single day in order to function correctly and when you restrict it too much, or take that nutrition away, poor health will quickly kick in, robbing you of your energy, causing you to look older than you are, and actually stalling weight gain. These are the more positive of the terrible effects, because it will also affect your sleep, cause you to be deprived of focus and concentration, as well as putting too much strain on your heart and immune systems. Put simply, starvation is not something you should even consider. Eat when your eating window begins and stop eating when it closes. It's that simple.

With all the general intermittent fasting information delivered to your door, it's now time to get a little more specific. In our next chapter we're going to talk about the 16:8 method, something we've hinted towards a few times already. This is the method of choice for many people, and one which fits in with a general lifestyle very easily.

Again, before you embark on this, double check with your doctor to ensure you don't have any contraindications, but on the whole, you should be able to look forward to a new lifestyle change, one which will help you lose weight, feel more alert and healthy, and not cause you the hungry, agitation, and upset that perhaps many other low calorie, fad diets have in the past.

Let's check out the 16:8 method!

Chapter 2: Introducing The 16:8 Method

If you do any research into intermittent fasting methods, and there are quite a few, you'll find that the 16:8 method comes up first on most lists. You might also see this written as Lean Gains, but it is one and the same thing.

The 16:8 method is an intermittent fasting type, and it comprises of a cycle of fasting and eating normally. When following the 16:8 method you are not told that you cannot eat certain foods, and you're not told that you should eat specific foods either. The choice is yours and that means you have freedom to change up your eating habits according to what suits you. Of course, this does not mean that you can go around eating all the unhealthy foods simply because the diet doesn't specify! Moderation is something you need to exercise at all times, and something which will become far easier as you start to notice weight loss.

Weight loss is a cumulative effect in so many ways. When you see changes in your body and you see the scales start to change, you'll want to keep up the good work and momentum. That means you're far less likely to 'fall off the wagon' and opt for something unhealthy, and you will start to feel far better for kicking out the unhealthy foods too. You'll notice that your body feels better when you eat healthy fruits and vegetables, when you choose whole grains over white breads, white rice, etc, and you'll feel far less sluggish for not eating chocolate, crisps, and carb-laden foods. Of course, you can treat yourself occasionally, but the chances are you won't want to!

You see, healthy lifestyles actually become quite addictive!

What is The 16:8 Method?

Now it's time to get into the real nitty gritty of what this method actually entails.

We've mentioned that there are many different types of intermittent fasting, and some do actually ask you to fast for 24 hours, a few times a week. The 16:8 method differs because there are no long and arduous fasts, you simply fast for 16 hours every day, and eat normally for 8 hours.

Now, that sounds a lot, 16 hours, but you are going to be sleeping for most of it! You see, you can move the fasting period to suit your needs. We'll talk about how to follow the method in more detail shortly, but a good example is someone who needs to eat breakfast versus someone who doesn't specifically want to eat early in the mornings. We're all different, but most of us fall into one of these two categories. You might wake up staving hungry and need breakfast otherwise you can't focus, or you might wake up and simply need a coffee, and you feel a little sick if you eat straight away.

There are two ways you can manage this, just to give you an example of what the 16:8 method looks like.

If you need breakfast, you can eat it as soon as you wake up, kickstarting your 8-hour eating period. So, if you wake up at 8am, you have breakfast at 8.30am, and that means you need to finish eating by 4.30pm. You might go to bed at 10pm, which means you're only consciously fasting 5.5 hours. As you can see, it's not as horrendous as it sounds, and you can drink water, non-calorie containing drinks, and unsweetened, black tea or coffee during your fasting times too. It's actually highly recommended that you drink plenty of water anyway, because dehydration is not something you want to play Russian roulette with!

The other scenario is that you are someone who doesn't really want to eat when they wake up. In that case, you can get up, get dressed, have a black, unsweetened coffee, and you can skip breakfast, starting your eating window at lunch time. So, for instance, you would begin eating at 12pm. This means you can eat freely until 8pm. You would then perhaps sleep at 10pm, which means you're effectively not consciously fasting too much!

This is why the 16:8 method is so popular.

Of course, during your 8-hour eating window you need to be mindful of what you're eating. If you cram those 8 hours full of crisps and choc-olate, then you're going to eat far more calories than you should in the full 24 hours of the day, and you're probably going to gain weight, rather than lose it! If however you're mindful of what you eat, not particularly being restrictive, but simply thinking more along the lines of health, you'll be full and satisfied by the end of your eating window and read for your fast. This means you will lose weight quite easily and grab the overall benefits of intermittent fasting too.

Can you see how easy it can actually be? You might wonder if you are actually going to be able to have the main benefits we talked about in our last chapter if you're not really putting yourself under huge strain, e.g. you're not fasting for days straight, but the answer is yes! You are still fasting; you're just doing it subconsciously for the most part. This doesn't matter in terms of the benefits, because they'll still come your way - fasting is fasting!

Why is This Method Best For Beginners

The 16:8 method is one of the easiest to follow and easiest to understand, which is why many beginners choose it. Of course, it doesn't suit everyone and because one size doesn't fit all, it might be that some people switch to a different method after a short amount of time. That's fine, and that might be something you want to think about. We're going to cover some alternative methods a little later in the book, so always bear in mind that if you find the 16:8 method isn't working as well as you want it to, for you, then there are other alternatives.

For the most part however, the 16:8 method, or Lean Gains, is very successful for many, and it is a method which encourages healthy eating without rules and regulations in terms of restriction. There are no massive changes to lifestyle, which is something which many people struggle with when they try a different eating routine, e.g. the Keto Diet, Atkins, Paleo, etc. These all come with a lot of rules and regulations and there are lists of what you can and can't eat, and how it should be prepared. This can overwhelm many a beginner and cause them to rebel against it and say: 'no thanks!' The

16:8 method, and many other intermittent fasting methods, don't come with those rules attached. There is no weighing or counting required, simply making healthy decisions, which aren't rocket science. For example:

- Pizza is bad, brown bread is better
- Chocolate is bad, fruit is better
- Cakes are bad, vegetables are good

Can you see how easy it is? It's not rocket science to make healthy choices, and that doesn't mean you have to be 100% healthy all the time! Want a burger? Have one, but only once a week, and make sure the rest of that day is packed with healthy foods.

The other plus point is that the 16:8 method doesn't have to bother your social life. Most people want to head out with friends or their partner for dinner on occasion, or perhaps out for a few drinks, but this can be very difficult when following a low calorie or fad diet. With the 16:8 method, all you need to do is ensure that you schedule the get-together for your eating window. This might be more difficult if you're starting your eating window early and finishing early, but you can always meet up for lunch instead of dinner! There aren't restrictions on what you can eat, but in most restaurants, you can always make healthy choices on the regular menu. If your eating window finishes a little later, that means you have more scope in terms of time.

Let's sum up the main reasons why most beginners opt for the 16:8 method.

- It's easy to follow and doesn't require any counting, weighing, or monitoring
- You can alter your eating time according to your needs
- You can set much of your fasting period into your sleeping period, so you don't notice it quite so much

- The eating method doesn't need to interfere with your social life too much at all
- You are not restricted on what you can eat, provided you make sensible, generally healthy choices
- It doesn't feel like a diet, it feels more like a new lifestyle with timings, rather than food you can and can't eat
- You can still have calorie free drinks, water, and unsweetened, black tea or coffee
- You won't notice hunger quite so much with this type of eating plan, as there are no extremely long fasts involved

How to Follow The 16:8 Method

The 16:8 method is very flexible, and that means you can choose your own specific 8 hour eating window, according to your day. You might work shifts, and that means you sleep at different times. What you should do in that case is pick an 8-hour window which is when you are mostly awake. Obviously!

For example, if you are working nights and you are sleeping between the hours of 10am and 6pm, that means you can eat from 6pm until 2am. You would then probably be working until the following morning, when you would head off to sleep, but you could drink coffee (unsweetened and black) to keep you going also, and plenty of water. This might not work for you, so you could think about shifting your pattern and starting it later, perhaps if you don't feel like eating the moment you open your eyes. You could then choose an eating window of 9pm and eat freely until 5am.

It's really up to you!

We've already covered the two main methods most people try with the 16:8, and that is the skipping breakfast and starting to eat at lunch time routine, or in the case of someone who really needs breakfast because they can't concentrate without it.

It's not only about the when you can eat, it's about what you eat too. Whilst there are no restrictions and no lists of foods you must eat and foods you shouldn't, always remember that if you suddenly pile a huge breakfast or lunch on your plate after fasting, you're going to end up with stomach ache. That could mean that you end up eating too many calories within your eating window and actually put weight on, or you end up with stomach disturbances for the rest of your eating window, don't get enough fuel during that time because your stomach is so bloated you can't bear to eat, and then you're hungry during your fasting time. It's about choosing carefully, which we'll talk about a little more shortly.

So, how many calories should you eat? It depends on whether you want to lose weight or maintain. A standard calorie amount to maintain weight is 2500 calories per day for a man, and 2000 calories per day for a woman. This does depend on the height, current weight, and metabolism of the person, and is really only an average, healthy amount. If you want more solid guidelines on your specific circumstances, speak to your doctor, who will be able to give you a calorie aim plan tailored to your needs.

Within that calorie amount you should make sure that you get a good, varied diet. That means proteins, carbs, fats, vitamins and minerals. Again, we're going to cover what you can and can't eat, loosely because there are no rules, shortly, but varied is the way to go. Ironically this will also help you enjoy your new lifestyle more, because you're not bored and eating the same things all the time. This is a pitfall many people suffer with regular low-calorie diets; the change is so restrictive that they end up eating the same thing day in, day out, and over time they get so bored and simply rebel against it. This usually ends in a binge day which causes extreme guilt and then leads them to throw the diet in the bin and go back to eating whatever they want.

Whilst following the 16:8 method you should also make sure that you drink plenty of water throughout the day, whether fasting or eating. This ensures that you don't become dehydrated and will also aid in digestion. In addition, you should also exercise too!

Now, there are no rules to say that you must exercise whilst following an intermittent fasting routine, but it will help you lose weight faster, and it will help with your general health and wellbeing. Exercise is fantastic on so many levels, not least helping to build lean muscle, which also boosts your ability to burn fat as an energy source. Exercise is also known to help with mental health issues, such as anxiety and depression, as well as stress. We all live stressful lives, and a little exercise can sometimes be enough to reduce it to levels which are extremely manageable. Aside from anything else, exercise can be a sociable and fun activity!

So, let's sum up how to follow the 16:8 method quickly.

- Eat for 8 hours per day, consecutively - you cannot break these hours up, they must be observed as one block of time
- Fast for 16 hours per day, again, this needs to be done consecutively
- You can choose when you take your 8-hour eating block, but it's a good idea to stick to the same times every day, so your body gets into a routine
- Your fasting times should coincide with sleeping, to cut down on the amount of conscious fasting
- Do not be afraid to miss breakfast, in this eating routine, there is no 'important meal of the day', there is simply an important eating window
- You can drink unsweetened, black tea and coffee, water, and other non-calorie containing drinks freely throughout your eating and fasting times, and you should certainly consume

enough water throughout the day to ensure you don't become dehydrated

- During your eating period, you should spread your meals out carefully, so you don't 'binge' when you initially break your fast. This will only lead to stomach aches and other unpleasant gastric symptoms!

- Choose healthy meals as much as possible, but there are no restrictions on what you can eat. If you go unhealthy however, remember that you're not going to create the calorie deficit required for weight loss

- Whilst you don't need to count calories whilst following the 16:8 method, it's worth bearing the standard calorie amounts in mind, which is 2500 for a man and 2000 for a woman, every day, as an average

- You should also exercise if you want to gain extra health benefits and speed up weight loss also

- Never be tempted to cut down your eating window or to restrict your calorie amount beneath the average - this will lead you towards extreme hunger and also borderline starvation is you refuse to eat. Remember, fasting is not starving!

What You Can And Can't Eat

Again, there are no rules on what you can eat and what you can't eat, it's totally free choice when following the 16:8 diet. What you should bear in mind however is overall health and choices which are considered healthy, compared to unhealthy.

The idea is to create that calorie deficit during the full 24-hour span. You do this by ensuring that you fast and eat for the correct ratios of time, e.g. 8 hours eating and 16 hours fasting, and that during your eating times you stick to healthy options as much as possible. You will feel infinitely better as a result also.

If you want a few ideas on some of the healthiest foods you can incorporate into your day generally, check out the list below.

- Eggs - Make sure you eat the yolk because this contains the vitamins Nd protein!
- Leafy greens - We're talking about things like spinach, collards, Kale, and Swiss chards to name a few, and these are packed with fiber and low in calories too
- Oily and fatty fish, such as salmon - Salmon is a fish which will keep you feeling full, but it's also high in omega 3 fatty acids which are ideal for boosting brain health, reducing inflammation, and generally helping with weight loss too. If salmon isn't your bag, try mackerel, trout, herring, and sardines instead
- Cruciferous vegetables - In this case you need to look toward Brussels sprouts, broccoli, cabbage, and cauliflower. Again, these types of vegetables contain a high fiber amount which help you feel fuller for longer, but also have cancer fighting attributes

- Lean meats - Stick to beef and chicken for the best options, but make sure that you go for the leanest cuts possible. You'll get a good protein boost here, but you can also make all manner of delicious dishes with both types of meat!
- Boiled potatoes - You might think that potatoes are bad for you, and in most cases, they are, especially if you fry them, but boiled potatoes are actually a good choice, especially if you're lacking in potassium. They are also very filling.
- Tuna - This is a different type of fish to the oily fish we mentioned earlier, and it's very low fat, but high in protein. Go for tuna which is canned containing water and not oil for the healthiest option. Pile it onto a jacket potato for a delicious and healthy meal!
- Beans and other types of legumes - These are the staple of any healthy diet and are super filling too. We're talking about things like kidney beans, lentils' Nd black beans here, and they're high in fiber and protein.

- Cottage cheese - If you're a cheese fan, there's no reason to deny yourself, but most cheeses are quite high in fat. In that case why not opt for cottage cheese instead? This is high in protein and quite filling, but low in calories.

- Avocados - The fad food of the moment is actually very healthy and great for boosting your brain power! Mash it up on some toast for a great breakfast packed with potassium and plenty of fiber.

- Nuts - Instead of snacking on chocolate and crisps, why not snack on nuts? You'll get great amounts of healthy fats, as well as fiber and protein, and they're filling too. Don't eat too many however as they can be high in calories if you overindulge.

- Whole grains - Everyone knows that whole grains are packed with fiber and therefore keep you fuller for longer, so this is the ideal choice for anyone who is trying intermittent fasting. Try quinoa, brown rice, and oats to get you started.

- Fruits - Not all fruits are healthy, but they're certainly a better option than chocolate and crisps! You'll also get a plethora of different vitamins and minerals, as well as a boost of antioxidants into your diet - ideal for your immune system.

- Seeds - Again, just like nuts, seeds make a great snack, and they can be sprinkled on many foods, such as yogurt and porridge. Try chia seeds for a high fiber treat, whilst being low calorie at the same time.

- Coconut oil and extra virgin olive oil - You will no doubt have heard of the wonders of coconut oil, and this is a very healthy oil to try cooking with. Coconut oil is made up of something called medium chain triglycerides, and whilst you might panic at the word triglycerides, these are actually the healthy type! If you want to go for something totally low in calories however, then you can't beat extra virgin olive oil.

- Yogurt - Perfect for a gut health boost, yogurt is your friend because it will keep you full and it also has probiotic content, provided you go for products which say 'live and active cultures' on the pot. Avoid the overly sugary yogurt treats and anything which says 'low fat' normally isn't as positive as it sounds!

There are plenty of delicious foods to try there and you can easily create some tasty recipes with any of those ingredients! We're going to run you through some recipes a little later in the book, so you can see how easy healthy eating can be, and how satisfying too.

So, what shouldn't you eat? There is nothing that is off limits, but it's about how much of it you eat. If you want a slice of pizza, you can have a slice of pizza, but make sure you only have one and that you have a healthier diet for the rest of the day. Remember, one of the reasons why intermittent fasting is so popular is because it doesn't wag its finger at you when you grab a chocolate bar once in a while. You don't have to feel guilty because you gave in to a burger craving once in a week, provided you know that moderation has to stand in the middle of it all.

What is moderation exactly? It's knowing when to stop and knowing what is enough and what is too much. For instance, enjoying pizza in moderation could mean having a couple of slices of pizza once a week. You still get to enjoy what you like, but you don't have it all the time. Similarly, moderation is stopping at two glasses of wine, rather than drinking the bottle. It basically means you still get what you want, but you don't go OTT.

Summing up The 16:8 Method

Now you know what the 16:8 method is, do you think it is the method of choice for you? The only way to find out is to try it! If you try and you find it doesn't work for you, that doesn't mean that you've failed or that intermittent fasting isn't going to work for you overall; what it means is that another method might suit you better. In that case, you can try one of the other methods we're going to talk about a little later in the book.

Earlier on we mentioned about the possible downsides of intermittent fasting, and from reading about the 16:8 method you'll see that most of those are side-stepped with this particular eating routine. Women will also find that their hormones aren't affected as much, because there is no huge fasting period, and for the most part, you're sleeping through it too! You can also pick when you want to eat (provided the 8 hours are together), to fit in with your lifestyle. This means if you work nights, or you work shifts, this isn't an issue, and if you want to go out to eat with friends, you can do so, provided it is scheduled into your regular eating window.

Fasting for 16 hours sounds a lot, and it is, in fact it's more than half of your entire day if you take 24 hours as a whole, but you're also sleeping for around 8 hours of it anyway. That means that in effect, you're only consciously fasting for 8 hours, and those are times you'll probably be full anyway, e.g. in the evenings when you've had dinner and you're full, or in the mornings when you don't feel like eating. Put simply, the 16:8 method makes it feel like you're not fasting at all, and that's why so many people choose to follow it as a beginner's option.

You'll hear the 16:8 method called Lean Gains, but there is no major difference. The only slight difference is that Lean Gains, as the name suggests, really advocates the use of lean foods. If you're opting for a healthy lifestyle anyway, that should be a no brainer!

Provided you drink plenty of water whether fasting or eating, that you eat a healthy diet as much as possible, you hit your calorie average intake, and you exercise if you can, you'll find that weight loss is a given, as well as overall health and wellbeing. You'll feel full of energy, you'll find your sleeping pattern rights itself, you'll focus and concentrate far easier, you'll look better as a result of all these major gains, and you'll find the scales moving at the same time.

Now we've delved into what intermittent fasting is and we've talked about one of the easiest ways to go about it, it doesn't seem quite so scary after all, does it?

Chapter 3: Sample Three Week Meal Plan

By getting onto chapter 3, we're going to assume that you're seriously considering following the 16:8 method of intermittent fasting - great choice!

We've talked about how to follow it, what you should be eating, what you should probably avoid, and we've covered moderation, but nothing cements understanding like seeing it written down and shown in a hard example. That is what this chapter is going to do. We're going to talk you through a three week long meal plan on the 16:8 intermittent fasting method. Remember, this is not a hard and fast meal plan that you absolutely must follow to the letter, because the idea of intermittent fasting is that you have the element of choice. If you fancy a burger, go for it, just make sure you don't continue the bad eating choices for the rest of that day, and don't repeat it in the coming days!

It also depends on whether you're male or female, your starting weight, and your height as to how many calories you actually need to consume on a daily basis. For that reason, we can't be 'one size fits all'. What we will do however, is show you a three weeks' eating plan that sticks to the healthy averages.

This isn't something you have to stick to, it's something you can look at and gain inspiration from, and really cement your knowledge from. Of course, if you look at the plans and think they look delicious (which they are), then go for it and follow them as you please! Remember to drink plenty of water whether fasting or not, and also remember that it's up to you to ascertain which hours you're going to fast throughout and which you're going to eat throughout. That is not something we can pinpoint here, as it's a totally personal choice, depending upon your needs, preferences, and circumstances.

We should also point out that in this meal plan we've avoiding calling meals breakfast, lunch, and dinner. That is because you might not eat breakfast, and you might not start eating until lunch! We'll call them meal 1, 2, 3, etc. just for argument's sake, but remember, you don't have to eat in a specific way, it's just simply advisable to eat specific meals because that way your nutritional content is spread out across the eating window evenly.

Let's get started!

Week 1

Monday

Meal 1 - Egg and vegetable omelette with cheese. You can add whatever vegetables you like!

Meal 2 - Mashed avocado on toast with a boiled egg on the side

Meal 3 - Chicken stir-fry, with as many other vegetables as you want to add and noodles

Snacks - Apple with peanut or almond butter

Tuesday

Meal 1 - Porridge sprinkled with chia seeds and berries

Meal 2 - Scrambled eggs with two slices of grilled bacon and a grilled tomato

Meal 3 - Meatballs made with whatever lean meat you like, covered in tomato sauce and served with wholegrain spaghetti

Snacks - Yogurt

Wednesday

Meal 1 - Low fat pancakes with one spoon of Nutella and berries

Meal 2 - Vegetable soup

Meal 3 - Grilled salmon served with vegetables and quinoa

Snacks - Fruit salad

Thursday

Meal 1 - Strawberry and banana smoothie

Meal 2 - Chicken salad (grilled or steamed chicken)

Meal 3 - Jacket potato with chili con carne (made with lean mince) and salad

Snacks - A handful of nuts and an apple

Friday

Meal 1 - Scrambled eggs with sautéed mushrooms

Meal 2 - Soup of your choice

Meal 3 - Homemade pizza topped with vegetables

Snacks - Apple and peanut butter

Saturday

Meal 1 - Breakfast frittata

Meal 2 - Boiled eggs and salad

Meal 3 - Chicken casserole

Snacks - A couple of squares of dark chocolate

Sunday

Meal 1 - Mushroom omelette with a little cheese

Meal 2 - Smoked salmon wrap

Meal 3 - Chicken drumsticks, rice and salad

Snacks - Keto-style garlic bread

Week 2

Monday

Meal 1 - Bacon and eggs - Remember, grill the bacon and fry eggs in olive oil!

Meal 2 - Caesar salad

Meal 3 - Homemade lasagna

Snacks - Chocolate covered nuts (a handful only)

Tuesday

Meal 1 - Scrambled eggs with smoked salmon

Meal 2 - Nicoise salad with tuna

Meal 3 - Homemade chicken curry

Snacks - Yogurt

Wednesday

Meal 1 - Caprese omelette

Meal 2 - Chicken and yogurt kebabs

Meal 3 - Beef stuffed portobello mushrooms

Snacks - Fruit salad

Thursday

Meal 1 - Fruit of your choice smoothie

Meal 2 - Shrimp salad

Meal 3 - Slow cooked beef stew

Snacks - Pineapple chunks

Friday

Meal 1 - Porridge with a berry topping

Meal 2 - Vegetable quesadilla

Meal 3   Homemade chicken fajitas with wholegrain wraps (more than two)

Snacks - Homemade strawberry mousse

Saturday

Meal 1 - Rutabaga fritters and grilled bacon

Meal 2 - Tuna and egg salad

Meal 3 - Chicken wings in cheese and broccoli sauce

Snacks - A handful of nuts

Sunday

Meal 1 - Eggs Benedict

Meal 2 - Turkey salad

Meal 3 - Roast chicken, 'Sunday dinner'

Snacks - A couple of squares of dark chocolate

Week 3

Monday

Meal 1 - Salami and brie cheese plate

Meal 2 - Chicken noodle soup

Meal 3 - Homemade moussaka

Snacks - Carrot sticks

Tuesday

Meal 1 - Bacon and onion frittata

Meal 2 - Chicken and avocado salad

Meal 3 - Meatloaf and green beans

Snacks - Whichever fruit is in season, e.g. strawberries, cherries, etc.

Wednesday

Meal 1 - French toast, Keto-style

Meal 2 - Chicken soup

Meal 3 - Zucchini lasagna

Snacks - Chia seeds

Thursday

Meal 1 - Mushroom and bacon breakfast casserole

Meal 2 - Vegetable soup

Meal 3 - Chili con carne and rice

Snacks - Yogurt

Friday

Meal 1 - Mashed avocado on toast

Meal 2 - Baked eggs with tomatoes and peppers

Meal 3 - Shepherd's pie with a difference - make the topping with cauliflower instead of potato!

Snacks - One banana

Saturday

Meal 1 - Poached egg on toast

Meal 2 - Asian beef salad

Meal 3 - Spaghetti in tomato sauce

Snacks - Skinny (low fat) hot chocolate

Sunday

Meal 1 - Pancakes with grilled bacon, and a little maple syrup

Meal 2 - Small jacket potato with salad and a little cheese

Meal 3 - Goulash

Snacks - One scoop of frozen yogurt

Now you've had a look at just how well you can eat on the 16:8 method, can you see why so many people try it? Of course, this isn't restricted to this particular intermittent fasting method, as many of the other methods all allow you to eat quite freely, they just have different rules in terms of when to eat. Some days ask you to restrict your calorie intake, and some ask you to fast completely for a day. It depends on the method you choose as to the rules you need to abide by. In our next chapter we're going to talk about the various other types of intermittent fasting methods you might like to look into. Remember, it's personal choice which one you go for, because one size never fits all, but the 16:8 method is certainly one fo the easiest, because you get into a quick and easy routine from the get-go.

For completeness' sake, however, let's dedicate our next chapter to the various other intermittent fasting methods on offer.

Chapter 4: Other Intermittent Fasting Methods to Explore

As we just mentioned, this chapter is going to be about the various other types of intermittent fasting you might like to try. You don't have to start with the 16:8 method, you can start with any method you find yourself drawn to, and similarly, you might like to move away from the 16:8 method if you find it's not really giving you the effects you want.

The bottom line is that intermittent fasting is very rarely not 'for you', it's mostly about the method you choose. If one doesn't work, another probably will. As before, always check with your doctor before you start any type of intermittent fasting method, especially if you have any pre-existing medical conditions or you're on any type of medication. Aside from that, let's check out some of the other methods you might like to consider.

The 5:2 Diet, or Fast Diet

You will hear this particular intermittent fasting method called both the Fast Diet and the 5:2 method, but they are one and the same thing. This particular eating method was made famous by a British doctor called Michael Mosley and he went on to publish many articles and a book on the very same eating method.

Very similar to the 16:8 method, with the 5:2 method you will eat normally for five days of the week, i.e. nothing is restricted, and you simply need to keep general good health in mind. For the other two days of the week you need to restrict your calorie intake quite drastically, down to 500 calories for women and 600 calories for men. It's important to do these two low calorie days, to ensure the correct amount of weight loss comes your way.

You might wonder why this is considered a fasting method, because there is no actual fasting, i.e. abstaining from food, involved. That might be true, but this very low-calorie intake for two days of the week is enough to class it as fasting. This calorie intake is literally the bare minimum and it's vital that you don't go below these numbers otherwise you run the risk of making yourself ill. It's also important that you don't do more than two days at these levels. These two low calorie days should also not run consecutively, e.g. you shouldn't have your low-calorie days on a Friday and Saturday, or a Monday and Tuesday.

A sample routine for the 5:2 method could be:

• Monday - normal eating

• Tuesday - low calorie day

• Wednesday - normal eating

• Thursday - normal eating

• Friday - low calorie day

• Saturday - normal eating

- Sunday - normal eating

When you look at it like that, this isn't a particular difficult method, but the low-calorie days will be quite brutal at first and will lead to the risk of over-eating when your normal eating day starts. This is all down to willpower, and it is something you will need to try and develop in order to make this method work for you.

Pros:

- Five normal eating days per week with no restrictions, other than general healthy eating

- You can easily fit this method around your social life, by simply scheduling meals and days out when you have normal eating days

- You only need to really think about what you're doing for two days of the week

Cons:

- The temptation to overeat when you first start to eat normally after a low-calorie day can be overwhelming at first

- Low calorie days are going to be hard, especially when you first start

Eat, Stop, Eat Method

The Eat, Stop, Eat method is really, as the name suggests, a cycle of eating and then stopping which goes on throughout the week. You basically need to do one or two fasts per week, but these need to be for a full 24 hours at a time. For example, you would follow this possible routine:

- Monday - eat normally until 8pm and then begin your fast

- Tuesday - fast for a full 24 hours, i.e. you can start to eat at 8pm

- Wednesday - eat normally

- Thursday - eat normally

- Friday - eat normally

- Saturday - optional fast for a full 24 hours as before

- Sunday - eat normally

As you can see, if you do two full fasts, these are not consecutive and are spread out across the week. For many people, one fast is enough, but if you want to boost the effects then you might want to try two fasts over time.

The Eat, Stop, Eat method was made famous by Brad Pilon, a fitness expert and many people prefer it because it only involves one or two days of consideration, with normal eating for the rest of the time. Of course, normal eating also means healthy eating, and doesn't mean that you can eat whatever you want. As with the 5:2 method, the temptation to binge eat after a 24 hour fast can be very overwhelming and you will need to develop iron willpower to avoid this happening.

In addition, it's obviously very difficult to fast for a full 24 hours, so don't jump straight in and do two fasts per week; see how you go with one before making your decision.

Pros:

- You only need to fast for one or two times per week and the rest of the time you can eat what you want (within moderation and reason)

- You can choose either one or two fasts, depending on how you feel and what you can manage

- This method fits very well into your social life, because it only affects one or two days

Cons:

- Fasting for a full 24 hours is very difficult

- The temptation to binge eat after the full 24 hour fast will be very overwhelming and you will need to be very strong not to give in

Alternate Day Fasting

The name really gives this one away. Alternate day fasting basically means that you are going to fast every other day. You should never fast consecutively, and you should have one normal eating day in-between.

This method sounds brutal, but there are a couple of variations, and one is a little easier than the other. Overall however, alternate day fasting isn't the best option for first timers, and this is probably something to work up to if you want to give it a try. An alternate day fasting schedule could look something like this:

- Monday - normal eating
- Tuesday - 24 hour fast, or 500 calories only
- Wednesday - normal eating
- Thursday - 24 hour fast, or 500 calories only
- Friday - normal eating
- Saturday - 24 hour fast, or 500 calories only

• Sunday - normal eating

As you can see, even though the pattern doesn't work equally, you should never do two full fasts or restrictive days consecutively. Whether you opt for a full fast or a low-calorie day is up to you. 500 calories is, as we mentioned before, the very bare minimum, so the effects will be very similar whichever option you go for. You may find yourself feeling lethargic and tired when you first begin the alternate day fasting method, but this should clear as your body gets used to it, and the benefits kick in.

Pros:

• Guaranteed weight loss and many other benefits

• Normal eating days fit in well with your social life, provided you schedule everything on those days

• An easy schedule to follow, with one day on and one day off

Cons:

- Extremely difficult for beginners

- Fasts and low-calorie days will be very hard at first and the temptation to overeat when they end will be very overwhelming

The Warrior Diet

The Warrior Diet is another of the quite hard-core intermittent fasting methods and isn't one which is recommended for beginners. Any side effects of intermittent fasting are far more likely with this particular method, simply because it is so restrictive and cuts your eating window right down to the very bare minimum.

The Warrior Diet was originated by Ori Hof-mekler, a fitness expert and former member of the Israeli Special Forces who believes that we should eat according to ancient warrior stand-ards. This means fasting for the entire day and then eating a very large meal during the night time hours. This meal can be anything, and you're encouraged to eat, eat, eat.

During day time hours you are able to eat a few fruits and vegetables, provided they are raw, but nothing else, aside from fluids. Your eating window is only 4 hours in duration, and obviously the encouragement to eat whatever you want during just 4 hours can lead to stomach upsets unless you learn the types of foods to eat and which to avoid.

There are a few variations of the Warrior Diet in terms of how to lead up to it, as it's not recommended to jump straight in. However, the end result is the same and you will still end up fasting for 20 hours and eating for just 4.

Pros:

• Weight loss, pretty much guaranteed, and quite quickly

Cons:

- You will have to keep odd hours, as you must eat during the evening, before you sleep

- The chances of stomach disturbances at first are very high, and you need to learn the heavy foods to avoid and the lighter foods you should eat to avoid this

- Fasting for 20 hours is very hard, even when munching on raw vegetables and fruits

- The chances of side effects are far higher than any other intermittent fasting method

Spontaneous Meal Skipping

Many people do spontaneous meal skipping occasionally without even realizing it but making a conscious habit of it can actually turn into a very effective intermittent fasting method.

With the spontaneous meal skipping method you don't need to follow a specific plan, e.g. there are no 'do this on Monday', 'do this on

Tuesday' rules, and instead you have the free-dom and choice to control your day. This means you skip meals occasionally, e.g. when you simply don't feel hungry enough to eat, when you're busy, or you think it's a good time to do so.

We're programmed to believe that we need to eat three square meals every day otherwise we're going to end up poor of health and starv-ing. This isn't the truth. By reading about inter-mittent fasting to this point you should have learnt that the general rules don't apply. Pro-vided you get the right number of calories within 24-hour period, you are not going to starve, you're not going to avoid the right type of nutrition, and as a result, nothing detri-mental is going to occur. The body is perfectly able to go without food for an amount of time, so skipping a meal isn't going to be a problem. You simply need to monitor how you feel and eat something if you feel like you really need to, e.g. you feel very hungry genuinely, you're light-headed, shaking, etc.

In order to make this work, you need to do it on a regular basis, otherwise the effects aren't going to be cumulative. Whilst you don't need to plan spontaneous meal skipping, otherwise it's not spontaneous, your week could look something like this when you reflect back on it:

- Monday - You're not hungry so you skip breakfast, beginning to eat at lunch time
- Tuesday - You're a little busy for lunch, so you jump straight to dinner later in the day
- Wednesday - You eat normally
- Thursday - You wake up late, so you don't have time for breakfast
- Friday - You eat normally
- Saturday - You eat normally

- Sunday - You have a late breakfast and you're really full until dinner time, so you skip lunch and eat later

Of course, for the other meals you do eat, you should make sure you stick to generally healthy choices, otherwise you're simply eating the calories from the meal you missed, and you won't reap the benefits of fasting at all.

Pros:

- No need to plan anything out, you can be spontaneous and see how you feel on the day
- You have total control over your fasting and eating
- This is a very natural way to eat and fast

Cons:

- It can be easy to 'forget' to skip a meal, or not skip enough to make the effects noticeable

- You also need to eat healthy for the rest of the time otherwise you are simply eating the extra calories at a later time and you won't lose weight - you might even gain it!

- This may be a slower form of weight loss, because there is no specific plan in place; it depends on how dedicated you are to spontaneous skipping

Finding Your Ideal Method

These are the main intermittent fasting methods around currently, but because this is an ever-changing beast, and the dietary world is always shifting and changing, you can expect several more to rear their heads over time. With this in mind, you should always be open to new methods and learn about them, to see if they are suitable for you, or whether you want to stick with the method you've been following so far.

We're big advocates of the 16:8 method in this book, and really feel that is the best place to start for most people. However, with that being said, we also know that one size doesn't fit all, as we've said a few times so far. We've given you information on the other main types of intermittent fast, and some are easy to follow, some are more dedicated and therefore require extra effort. From this list, is there a different method that you think you would like to try first?

Remember, it's not a good idea to jump straight into alternate day fasting or The Warrior Diet, because these are method which are for advanced fasters and those who have an extremely high level of general health and fitness. Opting for these harder methods from the get-go, when you have no specific experience of fasting could lead you towards all manner of effects, such as digestive upsets, fatigue, low immunity, and extreme hunger. Of course, these effects will pass, but it's not worth putting yourself through the upset when there are just as effective ways, which won't cause you all these unwanted affects.

The 5:2, or Fast Diet, is probably the second easiest method to follow. Whilst the two low calorie days are hard, with only 500 calories for women and 600 for men, the other five days are normal and don't require any planning, other than general healthy eating. This may be another option if you find the 16:8 diet isn't quite rigorous enough, or it doesn't suit you. Spontaneous meal skipping is another good option, however it may not be structured enough for many people and could lead to a lack of results if not enough meals are skipped.

The best way to choose the ideal method for you is to think about what you can handle and what you're going to struggle with. It's okay to challenge yourself but remember that the whole point of intermittent fasting isn't just the weight loss and the other health benefits, but also the fact that it fits into a regular lifestyle far easier than a traditional low calorie or fad diet. When your intermittent fasting method starts to really interfere with your lifestyle, you know you should think about another option.

Remember, intermittent fasting is designed to be a sustainable, long term answer to health and wellbeing. If your method doesn't allow you to do the things you love, and eat the things you love (in moderation, of course) then that's a pretty hard and fast sign that you've chosen the wrong one. There are no rules that say you need to stick with the first method you choose. Whilst swapping from one method to another is going to confuse your body a little at first, everything will catch up within a few days, so if you do feel you want to change your method of choice, that's certainly something you can do, without any worries.

Goodbye, And Good Luck!

We're now at the end of our informational chapters and our final chapter is going to be a fun-filled example of the delicious food you can try when you're eating healthily, as part of an inter-mittent fasting routine, specifically the 16:8 method. We're going to give you a bonus of 20 delicious recipes that you can make from scratch. Remember, making food yourself is far better than buying it pre-packed, and if you choose the freshest, preferably organic produce, you'll get far more in the way of nutrients and general goodness.

Eating healthily doesn't have to be rocket sci-ence, and it certainly doesn't have to be difficult. You'll come to know which foods to eat and which to only enjoy in moderation as you fall into your method and it becomes a part of your life. Generally speaking, healthy eating should mean you follow these rules:

- Frying is bad, unless you use coconut oil or ex-tra virgin olive oil
- Grilling, boiling, broiling, and steaming is bet-ter than frying

- If you opt for butters or other fats, make sure you stick to minimal amounts, e.g. if you put butter on bread, scrape it on, and then scrape it off to remove the excess

- Lean meat is far better than meat which has a large fat content on it, and it's tastier

- Always go with meat which comes from a grass-fed animal

- Stick to organic and fresh produce, to avoid the use of pesticides and other additives

- Always go for free range eggs and dairy products, and avoid farm or cage products

- Any fish you purchase, check to see that it is mercury free, and fresh water caught, not farm reared

- Go for variation and make sure you don't eat the same thing a few times in a row - you'll only get bored and try and go for something unhealthy!

- If you think you're hungry, it's possible that you're not and you're simply bored or thirsty.

Try and distract your mind by reading a book, doing something, or going for a walk, and have a drink of water, to see if the feeing passes

- Real hunger is felt in the stomach, with rumblings known as pangs. False hunger is felt in the mouth or is a figment of your imagination. You'll learn to know the difference as you get into your fasting routine

- Exercise will make you feel lighter on your feet, full of energy, and far healthier, so make it a part of your routine, no matter what type of exercise you choose

- If you have a bad day and you reach for an unhealthy snack, do not beat yourself up. Simply vow not to allow it to snowball and go back to your healthy ways. You're human, after all!

Those are the loose rules you should live by. If you can do that, and you really embrace your new fasting lifestyle, you'll certainly notice the pounds falling off, and the health benefits coming your way.

All that's left to say, is good luck!

Chapter 5: BONUS: Delicious And Easy 16:8 Method Recipes

As our final gift to you, we're going to show you how to recreate 20 delicious recipes which you can easily incorporate into your 16:8 eating plan. No more being hungry, no more restrictions, these recipes are delicious, easy to make, and they won't break the bank either!

For most of the receipts you won't need any specific, or out of the ordinary cooking equipment. You will however need some food weighing scales, and tablespoon and teaspoons, as well as cups. These will help you weigh out the ingredients correctly, and therefore avoid you adding too much of something and either ruining the recipe so it doesn't work out correctly, or taking the health side of the recipe too far to one side, and making it unhealthy!

We're not going to give you specific meal names, e.g. breakfast, lunch, or dinner, because as we mentioned in our sample meal plan chapter, you might not eat breakfast, and you might decide to start eating at lunchtime! Intermittent fasting overall is about choice, so these recipes are going to be varied in terms of their bulk and content, so you can choose when you want to make them. Some can also be made ahead of time and placed in the freezer - again, intermittent fasting is designed to fit in with your lifestyle, so why not make batches and then defrost them when you plan to enjoy them, perhaps after work or after a busy day doing whatever it is you do!

You'll also notice that our recipes come complete with macros, and these are the measurements of nutrition within each recipe. For instance, how many calories, how much carb content, protein, fat, etc. This will help you choose which meals to make on specific days, so that you don't go too calorie heavy, or otherwise.

No more chat let's get down to business!

Chicken, Vegetable and Pesto Stir-fry

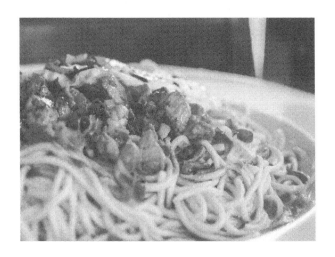

Serves 4

Preparation time - 10 mins

Cooking time - 20 mins

Macros per serving:

Calories 434

Carbs 18.5g

Fat 20g

Protein 8g

Ingredients

- 2 tbsps olive oil
- 6 boneless and skinless chicken thighs
- 2 sun-dried tomatoes, chopped roughly
- 4 asparagus spears
- 2 tbsps basil peso
- 8 cherry tomatoes, halved

Method

1. Preheat your stove to a medium heat
2. Take a large skillet pan and add the olive oil, allowing it to heat up
3. Once hot, add the chicken to the pan and sprinkle salt over the top
4. Take half of the sun-dried tomatoes and add them to the pan
5. Cook the contents of the pan for around 10 minutes, making sure you turn the chicken over every so often

6. Once the chicken is cooked, take it out of the pan along with the tomatoes, but leave the oil inside

7. Now, add the asparagus to the pan and add a little salt

8. Add the rest of the sun-dried tomatoes to the pan also and cook for another 10 minutes

9. Once cooked, place onto a serving plate

10.   Put the chicken back into the pan and stir in the pesto, cooking for a couple of minutes, ensuring the chicken is extremely hot

11.   Place the chicken onto the serving plate

12.   Serve with the cherry tomatoes on the side

Homemade Turkey Burger And Relish

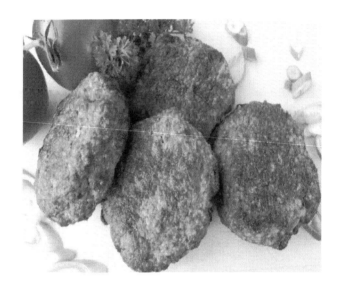

Serves 4

Preparation time - 10 mins

Cooking time - 20 mins

Macros per serving:

Calories 258

Carbs 10g

Fat 13g

Protein 3g

Ingredients

- 2lb ground turkey, made into four patties
- 1 onion, finely chopped
- 1 red bell pepper, chopped up finely
- 3 cups red cabbage, chopped or shredded
- 1 tbsp olive oil
- 0.25 cup balsamic vinegar
- 0.25 tsp garlic salt
- 4 lettuce leaves, large if possible

Method

1. Take a large skillet pan and place over a medium heat
2. Add the olive oil and allow it to reach temperature

3. Add the onion, red cabbage, and the pepper to the pan and cook until everything has softened

4. Now add the balsamic vinegar and the garlic salt and combine everything together, letting it simmer for a few minutes, until the contents have caramolized from the vinegar

5. Remove the contents of the pan and set aside to cool

6. Take your turkey patties and season with salt and pepper

7. Cook your patties for around 4 minutes on each side in either a pan or under the grill

8. Once cooked, transfer each patty onto a lettuce leaf and add some of the relish on top

Homemade Tuna Fish Cakes With Lemon Sauce

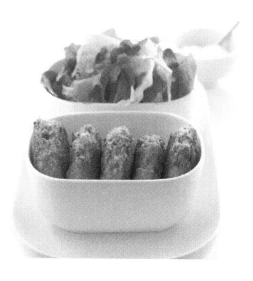

Serves 1

Preparation time - 10 mins

Cooking time - 20 mins

Macros per serving (2 cakes are one serving):

Calories 280

Carbs 14g

Fat 11g

Protein 4g

Ingredients

For the tuna cakes:

- Half a zucchini, grated

- 1 can of drained tuna

- 2 tbsp oats

- 2 tbsp cheese of your choice, shredded

- 1 egg

- 0.24 tsp garlic salt

- 0.25 tsp dill

- 0.25 tsp onion powder

For the sauce:

- 2 tbsp yogurt, Greek style is best

- 1 tsp juice of a lemon

- 0.25 tsp dill

- 0.25 tsp garlic salt

Method

1. Take a piece of cheese cloth, or similar and place the grated zucchini inside, twisting so that all the liquid comes out
2. In a medium bowl, place the drained zucchini inside and add the tuna, oats, shredded cheese, the garlic salt, dill, onion powder, pepper, and the egg, combining everything together well
3. Take a large frying pan and add a little olive oil, or cooking spray if you prefer
4. Take half of the mixture and form a ball, before flattening it into a fish cake style, repeating with the other half
5. Place the cakes into the frying pan, cooking over a medium heat for around 6 minutes on each side

6. Meanwhile, combine the sauce ingredients into a small mixing owl and ensure they are mixed together well
7. Once the fish cakes are cooked place them on a serving plate and allow to cool just slightly
8. Add a spoonful of the sauce on top and enjoy!

Healthy Breakfast Burritos

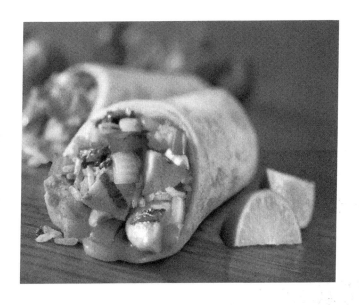

Serves 4

Preparation time - 5 mins

Cooking time - 10 mins

Macros per serving:

Calories 352

Carbs 22g

Fat 20g

Protein 8g

Ingredients

- 8 eggs
- 1 tbsp milk
- 1 tbsp garlic, minced
- 1 red pepper, minced
- Half an onion, red if possible, minced
- 4 slices of bacon, cooked
- Salt
- Pepper
- 4 tortilla wraps (multi-grain or wholegrain)
- A little cheese (optional)

Method

1. Take a medium sized saucepan and heat over a medium heat
2. Add the garlic and cook for a couple of minutes, until fragrant
3. Whisk the eggs with the milk and place to one side

4. Add the pepper and onion to the pan and allow to cook for a couple more minutes,

5. Add the eggs to the pan and cook for 4 minutes

6. Once cooked, add a quarter of the egg mixture onto each tortilla wrap and add one piece of the bacon on top

7. You can add cheese if you want, although it isn't necessary

8. Wrap up and enjoy!

Delicious Egg Casserole

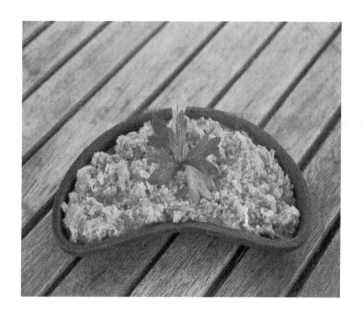

Serves 8

Preparation time - 10 mins

Cooking time - 30 mins

Macros per serving:

Calories 370

Carbs 23g

Fat 20g

Protein 24g

Ingredients

- 4.5 cups brown bread, cut into cubes
- 2 cups cheese, shredded
- 10 eggs, beaten
- 0.25 pint milk
- 1 tsp dry mustard
- 1 tsp salt
- 0/25 tsp onion powder
- 8 slices bacon, cooked and crumbled up
- 0.5 cup mushrooms, chopped

Method

1. Preheat your oven to 325C
2. Take a baking dish, around 13 inches in size and spray it with some cooking spray, to avoid sticking

3. Take the cubed pieces of bread and lay them in the bottom of the baking dish, evenly, so that the bottom is totally covered over

4. Add the cheese on the top, in one even layer

5. Take a separate mixing bowl and combine the milk, mustard, eggs, pepper, onion powder and the salt until completely mixed together

6. Add the mixture over the top of the bread and the cheese evenly

7. Now add the bacon and mushrooms on top, again making sure to stick to an even layer

8. Place the baking dish in the oven for half an hour. You will know when it is finished because it will have turned a wonderful golden brown

9. Remove from the oven and place to one side to cook for ten minutes

10.   Cut into slices and serve

Chicken Cobb Salad, With a BBQ Twist

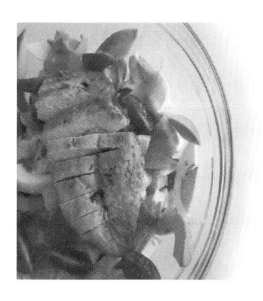

Serves 1

Preparation time - 10 mins

Cooking time - 25 mins

Macros per serving:

Calories 280

Carbs 19g

Fat 9.5g

Protein 27.5g

Ingredients

- 3oz chicken breast, no bones and no skin
- 2 tbsp BBQ sauce
- 2 slices bacon, chopped into small pieces
- 1.5 cups of romaine lettuce, chopped
- 0.25 cups cherry tomatoes, chopped
- 0.25 avocado, chopped
- 1 boiled egg, chopped

Method

1. Preheat your oven to 350C
2. Take the chicken and brush it with 1 tbsp of the BBQ sauce
3. Take a baking dish and spray with a little cooking spray

4. Place the chicken inside the baking dish and place into the oven for 25 minutes, or until the chicken is completely cooked through

5. Whilst the chicken is cooking, cook your bacon according to your preference and chop up once cooked

6. Take a serving bowl and place your romaine lettuce inside, arranging carefully

7. Add the chicken and bacon once cooked, as well as the egg, tomatoes, and the avocado

8. Drizzle the rest of the BBQ sauce over the top and enjoy whilst still warm

Hearty Quinoa And Carrot Soup

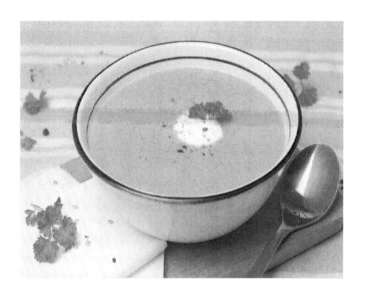

Serves 4

Preparation time - 10 mins

Cooking time - 50 mins

Macros per serving:

Calories 280

Carbs 44g

Fat 7g

Protein 9g

Ingredients

- 1 tbsp coconut oil

- 1 medium onion, chopped

- 1 small shallot, chopped very finely

- 1 tsp garlic, minced

- 1 tsp thyme, fresh is best in this case

- 3 sage leaves, chopped. Again, go for fresh if you can

- 1 tsp cumin

- 0.25 tsp turmeric

- A little black pepper, according to your preferences

- 1lb carrots, chopped

- 0.5lb parsnips, chopped

- 0.25 cup quinoa, uncooked and ensure it is rinsed out and drained thoroughly

- 5 cups broth, vegetable is best, or you can use simple water

Method

1. For this recipe you will need a large saucepan, or stock pot

2. Add the coconut oil and place over a medium heat

3. Once hot, add the garlic, onion, and the shallot and cook for around 6 minutes

4. Add the cumin, turmeric, thyme and the sage, with the pepper and combine well

5. Now add the parsnips and the carrots and stir once more

6. Add the quinoa and stir again

7. Add the broth or the water and allow the mixture to boil

8. Once the pan boils, turn the heat down to a simmer

9. Cook for 30-40 minutes, until everything is soft and cooked through

10. Take the pan from the heat and place it one side for around 5 minutes, until it has cooked down

11. You will now need an immersion or hand blander, so you can blend up the cup until it is smooth
12. Serve whilst still warm

Warming Lamb Stew

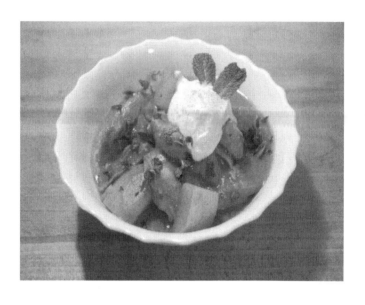

Serves 4

Preparation time - 15 mins

Cooking time - 1 hour 30 mins

Macros per serving:

Calories 343

Carbs 30g

Fat 9g

Protein 28.5g

Ingredients

- 2 tsp olive oil, extra virgin is best
- 1lb lamb, make sure it is as lean as you can get it, and cut into cubes
- A little salt
- A little pepper
- 1 large onion, chopped
- 1 celery stalk, chopped
- 2 garlic cloves, chopped
- 2 carrots, cut into small pieces
- 1.5 tsp oregano
- 2 cups broth, chicken broth works best here but you can use vegetable also
- 0.25 cup red wine, the dry version works well
- 1 x 15oz can of tomato sauce, the smoother the better
- 1 tsp zest from a lemon
- 0.5 tsp cinnamon
- 1 sweet potato, chopped

• 1 lemon, chopped

Method

1. You will need a Dutch oven for this recipe, and you need to add the oil and set to a medium to high heat
2. Once heated up, add the meat and add a little salt and pepper to your taste
3. Sear the lamb on both sides
4. Now, add the celery and the onion and cook for around 4 minutes, until soft
5. Add the garlic and cook for half a minute
6. Add the oregano and combine well, and then add the carrots, stirring all the while for another half a minute
7. Add the wine, the broth, the tomato sauce, the lemon zest, and the cinnamon and combine everything well
8. Next add the sweet potato and the lemon and combine once more

9. Allow the mixture to reach boiling point and then turn the heat down to a lower temperature, covering over and allowing to simmer
10. Cook until the vegetables are soft, and the lamb is totally cooked, for between 80-90 minutes
11. You may need to add more salt and pepper, according to your personal preferences

Spicy Chicken Marsala

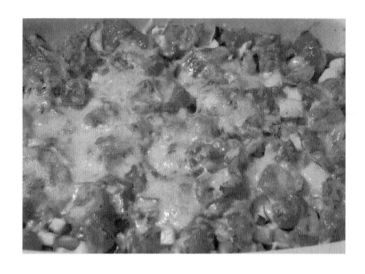

Serves 4

Preparation time - 10 mins

Cooking time - 20 mins

Macros per serving:

Calories 365

Carbs 18g

Fat 6g

Protein 51g

Ingredients

- 4 chicken cutlets, pounded until they are quite thin
- A little salt to taste
- 1 egg, beaten
- 0.5 cup of whole-wheat flour, plus another 1.5 tbsp
- 2 x 8oz packs of button mushrooms, sliced
- 4 cloves of garlic, minced
- 0.5 cup Marsala wine, the dry version works best
- 1 cup of chicken broth, low fat is best
- 0.25 cup of Greek yogurt
- A little black pepper
- Cheese for topping if you want to

Method

1. You will need two non-stick pans for this recipe, and they both need to be placed over a medium to low heat
2. Season your chicken with a little salt and wait for the pans to heat up, spraying with a little cooking oil
3. In a small mixing bowl, add the beaten egg and the 0.5 cup of whole-wheat flour and mix together
4. Dip the chicken into the mixture and cover completely, before placing into the pans, two in each
5. Cook the chicken for about 4 minutes on each side and then
6. Place the chicken onto a plate and keep warm with aluminum foil
7. Clean the pans out and turn the heat up, adding a little more spray to the pans
8. Place one package of mushrooms into each pan and cook for around 3 minutes

9. Now place all the mushrooms in one pan and add the garlic and a little salt

10. Turn the heat down and cook for one more minute

11. Add the rest of the whole-wheat flour to the mixture, along with the wine and the broth, combining everything well

12. Allow the mixture to simmer, for around 3 minutes

13. Take the pan off the heat and add the yogurt and a little more salt and pepper, stirring well

14. Remove the foil from the chicken and place on a serving plate, pouring the Marsala sauce over the top

15. Add a little cheese to melt on top if you like

Quick Ratatouille

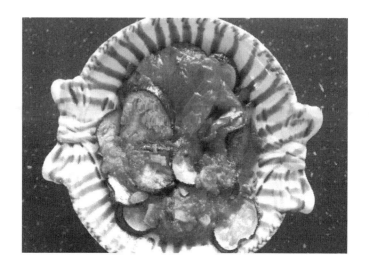

Serves 4

Preparation time - 10 mins

Cooking time - 12 mins

Macros per serving:

Calories 228

Carbs 3g

Fat 19g

Protein 3g

Ingredients

- 2 onions, sliced
- 4 cloves of garlic, chopped very finely
- 0.5 cup olive oil
- 1 green pepper, cut into small pieces
- 1 red pepper, cut into small pieces
- 1 aubergine (eggplant), cut into cubes
- 4 zucchinis, cubed
- 8 tomatoes, seeded and chopped
- 1 tbsp basil, shredded. Fresh is best but if you have to go with dried, just use 1 tsp)
- 1.5 tsp salt
- A little black pepper

Method

1. You will need a large and deep-frying pan or saucepan,

2. Add the oil and allow to reach a medium to high heat

3. Add the onions and the garlic and cook for a few minutes, until he onions are clear

4. Add the peppers, zucchini, and the aubergine (eggplant) and combine

5. Turn the heat down and play an over the pan, allowing it to simmer for around 10 minutes

6. Add the salt and pepper, as well as the tomatoes and stir well, covering the pan once more and allowing it to continue cooking for another 10 minutes

7. Take the lid off the pan and stir the mixture, allowing it to reduce

8. Add a little salt and pepper and serve whilst still warm. The mixture is done when it is blended well, but isn't particularly 'wet'

Cajun Chicken With Buckwheat Crust

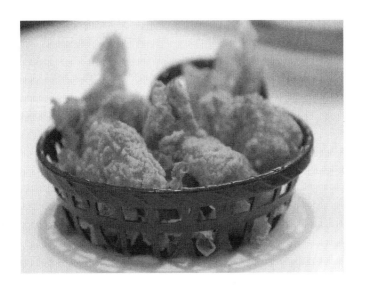

Serves 4

Preparation time - 10 mins

Cooking time - 20 mins

Macros per serving:

Calories 379

Carbs 9g

Fat 18g

Protein 45g

Ingredients

- 0.25 cup buckwheat flour
- 2 tbsp paprika powder, the sweet version is the best for this recipe
- 1 tsp turmeric powder
- 1 tsp cumin powder
- 1 tsp coriander powder
- A little salt
- A little pepper
- 0.5 tsp cinnamon powder
- A little coconut oil for cooking
- 4 chicken breasts, but you can use thighs if you prefer
- 1 red chili pepper, chopped very finely (be careful to wash your hands!)
- A few almonds, chopped very finely

Method

1. Take a mixing bowl and combine the flour and the powders
2. Take your chicken and coat evenly with the mixture
3. Take a large frying pan and add the coconut oil, allowing it to heat up over a medium to low heat
4. Place the chicken in the pan and cook on both sides until completely cooked through
5. Once cooked, transfer to a serving plate and serve with the finely chopped chili and the almonds
6. Add a little salt and pepper according to your personal preference

Healthy Mushroom And Arugula Pizza

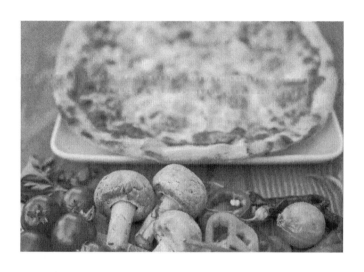

Serves 4

Preparation time - 10 mins

Cooking time - 20 mins

Macros per serving (one slice is a serving):

Calories 185

Carbs 4.5g

Fat 15g

Protein 7.5g

Ingredients

- Enough cornmeal to coat a 14" pizza pan
- 0.5lb wild mushrooms. You can go for a mix if you want to, including chanterelles, and porcini as some of the most flavorsome
- 2 tbsp olive oil
- A little salt and pepper
- 2 cups of arugula leaves, chopped roughly
- 1.5 tsp lemon juice, go for fresh for the best taste
- 1 cup grated cheese, Gruyere is ideal for this pizza
- 1 pack of pizza dough

Method

1. Preheat your oven to 260F
2. Take a 14" pizza pan and cover the base with the cornmeal evenly

3. Take an ovenproof dish and add 1 tbsp of the oil and the mushrooms

4. Add a little salt and pepper and stir everything to ensure it is evenly coated

5. Place in the oven for 10 minutes and then set aside

6. Take a mixing bowl and combine the lemon juice, the rest of the oil and the arugula, seasoning with salt and pepper

7. Next, make your pizza dough according to instructions and brush the edge with a little extra olive oil

8. Add the cheese on top of the dough evenly

9. Add the mushrooms, but make sure you leave around 2 inches towards the edge

10. Place in the oven for around 10 minutes

11. Once cooked, place to one side to cool for a couple of minutes

12. Cut into slices and place some of the arugula mixture on top

Easy Mexican Casserole

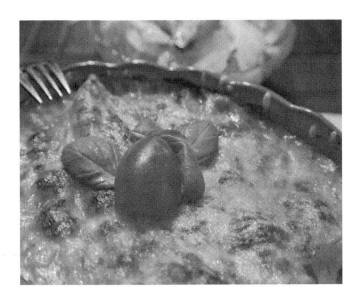

Serves 4

Preparation time - 15 mins

Cooking time - 45 mins

Macros per serving:

Calories 70

Carbs 4.5g

Fat 20g

Protein 4.6g

Ingredients

- 1 cauliflower head
- 0.5 onion, chopped
- 1 red bell pepper, chopped
- 1 green pepper, chopped
- 1 jalapeño pepper, chopped
- 1 tsp cumin
- 1 tsp chili powder
- 8 tomatoes, cherry work best, cut into halves
- 1.5 cups cheese, shredded

Method

1. Preheat your oven to 240C
2. Take a large skillet pan and heat up over a medium heat, with little olive oil
3. Add the onions, chili powder, cumin, and the upper and combine well, cooking for around 2 minutes
4. Remove from the heat and place to one side

5. Crumble the cauliflower up into small pieces and place in the microwave for around 3 minutes

6. Once finished, add the tomatoes and 1 cup of cheese and combine well

7. Add to the pepper mixture and combine once more

8. Take a medium baking dish and coat with cooking spray

9. Place the ingredients into the dish and spread evenly

10. Add the rest of the cheese and cook for half an hour

11. Allow to cool a little before slicing up and serving

Stuffed Portobello Mushrooms

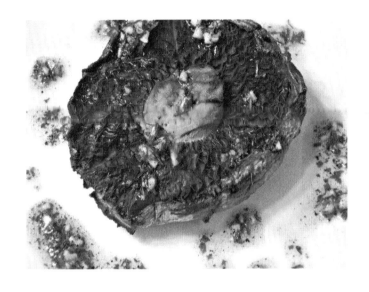

Serves 4

Preparation time - 10 mins

Cooking time - 20 mins

Macros per serving (2 mushrooms is one serving):

Calories 318

Carbs 11.6g

Fat 21.9g

Protein 21.6g

Ingredients

- 8 portobello mushrooms, the large ones are best
- 6oz kale, the fresher the better
- 8 slices of cheese, go for one you like best
- 2 tbsp olive oil, extra virgin is best here also

Method

1. Preheat your oven to 250C
2. Take a baking sheet and cover with parchment paper
3. Place the mushrooms onto the tray, with the 'cup' facing upwards
4. Drizzle a little of the olive oil over the top of the mushrooms and place in the oven for around 10 minutes
5. Once cooked, add a slice of cheese to each mushroom and a little of the cake

6. Place back in the oven for another 3 minutes; the mushrooms are cooked when the cheese is melted and bubbling
7. Allow to cool a little before serving

Quinoa And Turkey Stuffed Peppers

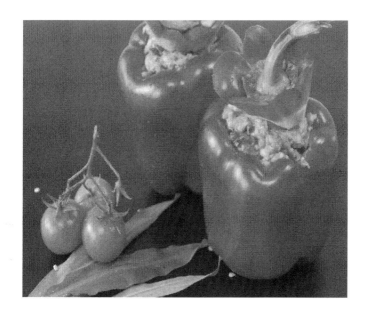

Serves 7
Preparation time - 5 mins
Cooking time - 55 mins

Macros per serving:
Calories 262
Carbs 22g

Fat 9g

Protein 23g

Ingredients

- 2 tbsp extra virgin olive oil

- 1 onion, red is best, diced

- 3 cloves of garlic

- 1 chipotle pepper, the larger the better, minced up

- 1lb lean turkey mince

- 1 tsp paprika, go for smoked if you can

- 1 tsp cumin

- 0.5 tsp salt

- 025 tsp black pepper

- 15oz fire roasted tomatoes, cut into small pieces

- 0.75 cup of drained black beans

- 0.75 cup of corn, frozen works well here

- 0.25 cup of cilantro, fresh if possible, diced

- 0.5 cup quinoa, dried

- 7 bell peppers, with the top cut off and de-seeded

- 0.75 cup cheese, shredded

Method

1. Preheat your oven to 240C
2. Take a saucepan and add a cup of water, allowing it to boil
3. Once the water boils, add the quinoa and cover over, bringing it to the boil once more
4. Reduce the quinoa down to a simmer, for around 12 minutes, before fluffing up and putting to one side
5. Take a large frying pan and add a little oil, setting over a medium to high heat
6. Add the diced onions and cook for around 3 minutes
7. Add the chipotle pepper and the garlic and cook for another minute

8. Add the paprika, salt, pepper, cumin, and the tomatoes, the cilantro, corn and the beans and mix everything together
9. Cook for around 5 minutes, until all the liquid has disappeared
10. Toss the turkey mince with the quinoa and add to the other ingredients, mixing to gether well
11. Take a large baking dish and spray with a little cooking oil
12. Place the peppers into the dish, making sure they won't fall over
13. Add the turkey mixture to the inside of each pepper
14. Place in the oven for 40 minutes
15. Add a little of the shredded cheese to the top of each pepper and place back in the of for another one minute
16. Once cooked, add the cilantro and serve

Light Fish Stew

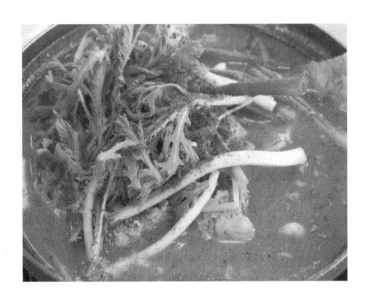

Serves 4

Preparation time - 10 mins

Cooking time - 25 mins

Macros per serving:

Calories 325

Carbs 26g

Fat 7g

Protein 34g

Ingredients

- 4 slices of brown bread cut into cubes. Make sure the bread is old, e.g. stale
- 2 tbsp olive oil
- 1 onion, chopped very finely
- 2 cloves of garlic, crushed and chopped
- 1 tsp chili flakes, dried
- 1 x 400g can of tomatoes, chopped
- 4 fillets of white fish, e.g. pollock or cod. You can use frozen here also
- 1 x 400g can of drained butter beans
- A little parsley, chopped

Method

1. Preheat your oven to 200C
2. Take a large baking sheet and add a little of the oil over the top
3. Arrange the bread onto the baking sheet and place in the oven for 10 minutes

4. Once cooked, place to one side

5. Take a large casserole dish (flameproof) and add the remaining oil, heating over a medium heat

6. Add the onions and allow to cook for around 10 minutes

7. Add the chili flakes and the garlic and combine, cooking for a further minute

8. Add the tomatoes and combine

9. Now add the fish and place a lid over the top of the dish

10. Simmer for 10 minutes, and then take the lid off

11. Add the butter beans and season with salt and pepper

12. Continue cooking until the fish is cooked and everything is soft

13. Add the bread pieces and serve with a little chopped parsley

Chili, Vegan Style

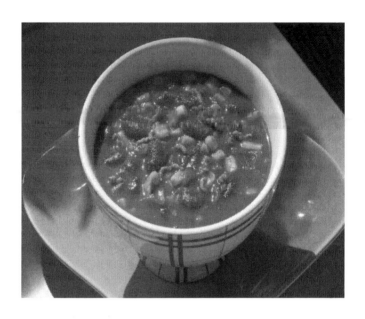

Serves 4

Preparation time - 15 mins

Cooking time - 45 mins

Macros per serving:

Calories 367

Carbs 48g

Fat 10g

Protein 12g

Ingredients

- 3 tbsp extra virgin olive oil
- 2 medium sized sweet potatoes, cubed
- 2 tsp paprika, the smoked version works best
- 2 tsp cumin, ground
- 1 large onion, chopped
- 2 carrots, chopped
- 2 sticks of celery, chopped
- 2 cloves of garlic, crushed and chopped
- 2 tsp chili powder, or less if you don't like it too spicy
- 1 tsp oregano, dried
- 1 tbsp tomato puree
- 1 red pepper, cubed
- 2 x 400g tins of tomatoes, chopped
- 1 x 400g tin of drained black beans
- 1 x 400g tin of drained kidney beans

Method

1. Preheat your oven 200C
2. Take a roasting tin and add 1.5 tbsp of the olive oil
3. Add the sweet potato to the tin, along with half the paprika and half the cumin
4. Mix everything together and season with a little salt and pepper
5. Place into the oven to cook for 25 minutes
6. Add the rest of the oil to a large pan and set over a medium heat
7. Cook the onion, celery and the carrot for around 10 minutes
8. Add the garlic and cook for a further minute
9. Add the tomato puree and the rest of the spices and combine everything, cooking for another minute
10. Add the chopped tomatoes and the red pepper, along with 200ml of warm water
11. Allow the chili to boil, and then turn the heat down to a simmer for 20 minutes

12.   Add the beans and combine, cooking for another 10 minutes

13.   Once the sweet potato is cooked, add that to the chili and combine

14.   Add a little salt and pepper and serve!

Citrus And Halloumi Salad

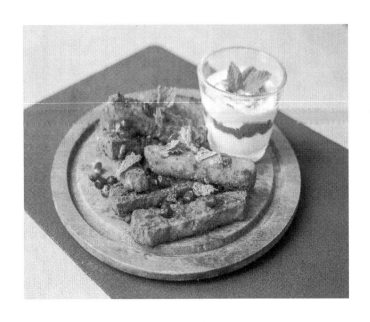

Serves 4

Preparation time - 5 mins

Cooking time - 15 mins

Macros per serving:

Calories 338

Carbs 15g

Fat 23g

Protein 16g

Ingredients

- 2 oranges

- 1.5 tbsp mustard, wholegrain works best

- 1.5 tsp honey

- 3 tbsp olive oil plus and an extra tbsp for cooking

- 1 tbsp white wine vinegar

- 2 carrots, peeled and cut into thin slices using a grater

- 1 x 225g of halloumi, cut into slices

- A handful of baby spinach or watercress

Method

1. Take the oranges and cut away the peel and the pith, cutting into segments, maintaining the juice in the bowl, and placing the segments to one side

2. Add the mustard, oil, vinegar and the honey and combine, seasoning a little if need be
3. Toss the carrots in the mixture
4. Take a medium sized frying pan and add a little oil, over a medium heat
5. Cook the halloumi on both sides until golden, for a few minutes
6. Meanwhile, toss the baby spinach or the watercress in the mixture and arrange on a plate
7. Add the halloumi on top and pour the mixture over the cheese, adding the oranges on the side

Pasta Bolognese Soup

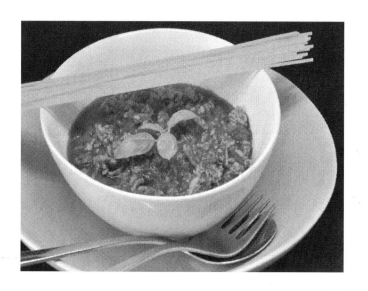

Serves 4

Preparation time - 10 mins

Cooking time - 35 mins

Macros per serving:

Calories 337

Carbs 35g

Fat 9g

Protein 24g

Ingredients

- 2 tsp olive oil
- 3 onions, chopped finely
- 2 carrots, peeled and chopped finely
- a celery stick, chopped finely
- 3 cloves of garlic, chopped finely
- 250g of lean steak/beef mince
- 500g passata
- 1 tbsp vegetable stock
- 1 tsp paprika, smoked works well
- 4 pieces of thyme, fresh
- 100mg penne, whole meal
- 45g parmesan cheese, grated finely

Method

1. Take a large pan and add the oil, heating over a medium heat
2. Add the onions and cook until translucent

3. Add the carrots, garlic, and the celery, cooking for 5 minutes

4. Add the mince to the pan and break it up well

5. Once the mince has browned, add the stock and the passata, adding 1 liter of hot water

6. Stir well and then add the thyme and paprika, combining once more

7. Add the lid to the pan and allow to simmer for 15 minutes

8. Add the penne and stir through, cooking for another 165 minutes

9. Add the cheese and stir

10.   Serve in bowls whilst still warm

Eggs With Avocado And Black Beans

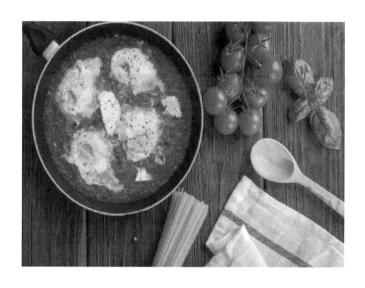

Serves 2

Preparation time - 5 mins

Cooking time - 5 mins

Macros per serving:

Calories 356

Carbs 18g

Fat 20g

Protein 20g

Ingredients

- 2 tsp olive oil
- 1 red chili pepper, sliced thinly
- 1 clove of garlic, sliced
- 2 eggs
- 1 x 400g tin of black beans, undrained
- 1 x 400g can of tomatoes, cherry if possible
- 0.25 tsp cumin seeds
- 1 avocado, cut into slices
- A little coriander, chopped

Method

1. Take a large frying pan and add the oil, allowing to heat over a medium to high heat
2. Add the garlic and the chili and cook until soft
3. Crack the eggs into the pan carefully

4. As the eggs begin to cook and set, add the whole contents of the can of beans into the pan, along with the tomatoes, mixing carefully

5. Add the cumin seeds

6. After a few minutes, remove the pan and add the avocado onto and a little coriander

7. Serve whilst still hot!

Made in the USA
Middletown, DE
30 May 2019